Health Technical Memorandum 2040

Design considerations

The control of legionellae in healthcare premises – a code of practice

London: HMSO

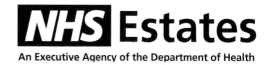
NHS Estates
An Executive Agency of the Department of Health

Cover photograph:
Scanning electron micrograph of a biofilm on latex showing
amoeba grazing the bacterial consortium (magnification x 1440).
Reproduced by kind permission of Julie Rogers and A B Dowsett,
Public Health Laboratory Service Centre for Applied Microbiology
and Research, Porton Down, Salisbury, Wiltshire.

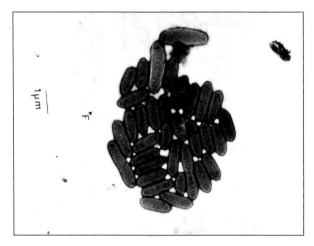

Above:
A colony of bacteria *Legionella pneumophila*. The bacteria are
non-sporing, typically 2–3 μm long, 0.3–0.9 μm wide. Flagella,
which can be clearly seen, provide mobility of the organism.
Reproduced by kind permission of Public Health Laboratory
Service Centre for Applied Microbiology and Research.

HMSO
Standing order service

Placing a standing order with HMSO BOOKS enables a
customer to receive future titles in this series automatically
as published. This saves the time, trouble and expense of
placing individual orders and avoids the problem of
knowing when to do so. For details please write to HMSO
BOOKS (PC 13A/1), Publications Centre, PO Box 276,
London SW8 5DT quoting reference 14 02 017.
The standing order service also enables customers to receive
automatically as published all material of their choice which
additionally saves extensive catalogue research. The scope
and selectivity of the service has been extended by new
techniques, and there are more than 3,500 classifications to
choose from. A special leaflet describing the service in detail
may be obtained on request.

About this publication

Health Technical Memorandum (HTM) 2040 provides recommendations, advice and guidance on controlling legionellae in healthcare premises. It is applicable to new and existing sites, and is for use at various stages during the inception, design, upgrading, refurbishment, extension and maintenance of a building.

HTM 2040 focuses on the:

a. legal and mandatory requirements;

b. design of systems;

c. maintenance of systems;

d. operation of systems.

It is published as five separate volumes, each addressing a specialist discipline:

a. **Management policy** – outlines the overall responsibility of managers of healthcare premises, and details their legal and mandatory obligations. It summarises the essential background information required to understand the principles of the control of legionellae. This is followed by an epidemiology of legionellosis, essential to understanding the rationale behind the various control and design measures advocated in succeeding volumes. A management checklist is provided in the Appendix to this volume; it lists the major tasks and should form the basis of a risk assessment;

b. this volume – **Design considerations** – highlights the overall requirements and considerations that should be applied to the design up to the contract document;

c. **Validation and verification** – considers the testing and commissioning aspects, also providing guidance on the identification of problem areas;

d. **Operational management** – considers aspects of preventing and controlling legionellae. It also contains information on the operation, maintenance and cleaning of evaporative cooling towers;

e. **Good practice guide** – gives advice on the course of action if an outbreak of legionnaires' disease is suspected, on the cleaning and disinfection of a cooling tower implicated in an outbreak of legionnaires' disease, and on the use of sodium hypochlorite solutions for chlorination of cooling water systems in hospitals. Further advice is given in respect of:

(i) emptying times for cooling tower ponds;

(ii) a questionnaire, to assess the serviceability of existing cooling systems;

(iii) a sample logbook for the planned maintenance of a cooling tower.

Guidance in this Health Technical Memorandum is complemented by the library of National Health Service Model Engineering Specifications. Users of the guidance are advised to refer to the relevant specifications.

The contents of this Health Technical Memorandum in terms of management policy, operational policy and technical guidance are endorsed by:

a. the Welsh Office for the NHS in Wales;

b. the Health and Personal Social Services Management Executive in Northern Ireland;

c. the National Health Service in Scotland Management Executive;

and they set standards consistent with Departmental Cost Allowances.

This HTM was written with the advice and assistance of experts in the NHS and industry.

References to legislation appearing in the main text of this guidance apply in England and Wales. Where references differ for Scotland and/or Northern Ireland these are given in marginal notes.

Where appropriate, marginal notes are also used to amplify the text.

Contents

1.0 Introduction

General

1.1 The guidance contained in this volume is applicable to new and existing sites, and is for use at various stages during the inception, design, upgrading, refurbishment, extension and maintenance of a building.

1.2 The approach should be to remove all potential sources of seeding, growth and spread of legionellae. Where this ideal cannot be achieved in existing situations, steps should be taken to control and prevent legionellae by sound operational management.

1.3 The control of legionellae is a continuing responsibility. The effectiveness of precautionary measures should be continually monitored and a continuing programme to ensure awareness should be devised. Although knowledge of legionellosis has improved markedly in recent years, there is a continuing misunderstanding about the method of dissemination. Many people are under the impression that cooling towers are the only source of legionellae in building service systems. All water systems are capable of colonisation by legionellae, and taps are just as capable of generating an aerosol as showers or, indeed, cooling towers.

1.4 The biggest risk is complacency, leading to the deterioration of water hygiene to the extent that an outbreak of the disease occurs.

1.5 Good practice design alone will not prevent outbreaks of legionellae.

1.6 The HTM does not include advice on water supplies for clinical equipment such as dialysers, nebulisers and respiratory humidifiers nor for sterile water services for pharmacy departments. Users of clinical humidifiers and nebulisers are reminded that sterile water, not tap water, should be used and they should be emptied and cleaned thoroughly following each period of use. All equipment with water reservoirs should be stored dry. Water for any purpose should meet functional and local requirements, but users must recognise that any water system may provide a suitable environment for legionellae and other water-borne organisms and should therefore be designed to take account of this.

2.0 Design considerations

General

2.1 The design and installation of the cold and hot water services in new, upgraded or refurbished NHS premises are required to comply with:

a. the local water undertaking's byelaws that are based on the Model Water Byelaws;

b. the Water Supply Byelaws Guide, published by the Water Research Centre (WRc) (ISBN 0-902156-71-3);

c. BS6700: British Standard Specification for design, installation, testing and maintenance of services supplying water for domestic use within buildings and their curtilages.

HTM 27 – 'Cold water supply storage and mains distribution' should also be consulted for guidance for the general design and operation of water systems in healthcare premises.

Scotland: SHHD/DS(80)26

2.2 If water for fire protection systems is stored in holding tanks these should be inspected and maintained regularly. If trace heating is used for frost protection, temperatures should be routinely checked for overheating.

2.3 While hose reels and other equipment may derive their water supply from the potable source, it is impracticable to maintain the wholesomeness of the water within such equipment. There is a risk that these water sources may become contaminated; all other water stored and distributed in healthcare premises should be treated as potable or wholesome, that is, fit for drinking.

2.4 All designs should aim to ensure that no water is stored or circulated at temperatures between 25 and 45°C. Cold water should ideally be below 20°C and hot water above 50°C. Special attention is needed where this ideal cannot be met. It should also be remembered that hot water above 45°C presents a scalding risk to some users. Taps or other outlets should not be installed if they will not be used regularly, that is, more than once per week.

2.5 Where taps are sited remotely and for practical purposes this cannot be avoided, they should be flushed through weekly for several minutes or until water temperature stabilises.

2.6 The WRc Water Fittings and Materials Directory should be consulted to identify approved products. As a general principle, traditional materials based on natural products such as linseed oil, jute or hemp support the growth of micro-organisms when used in water services; such materials are no longer permitted under the byelaws. Alternative materials vary in their ability to support microbial growth according to their chemical formulation and method of manufacture. Fittings and materials should be specified precisely, not by generic names.

Wet fire systems

2.7 Wet fire protection systems have been implicated in outbreaks of legionellosis. All hose reels and wet risers should be isolated from the potable water supply by a method permitted by the water byelaws. It should be noted that this does not give full protection but currently the balance of risk is in favour of preserving the performance of the fire safety systems. Further guidance will be issued when research has been completed.

Source water

2.8   Provided water is supplied from the public mains and its quality is preserved by correct design, installation and maintenance, it can be regarded as microbiologically acceptable for use without further treatment.

Northern Ireland: Equivalent provisions are proposed for Northern Ireland (Oct 93)

Scotland: The Private Water Supplies (Scotland) Regulations 1992

2.9   Private water supplies (bore holes and wells) are covered by the Private Water Supplies Regulations 1991 (Statutory Instrument No 2790).

Northern Ireland: Equivalent provisions are proposed for Northern Ireland (Oct 93)

Scotland: The Water Supply (Water Quality) (Scotland) Regulations 1990 with amendments

2.10   For design purposes it should be assumed that the water supply meets SI 1989 No 1147 – Water Supply, Water Quality Regulations of England and Wales. These regulations implement the European Commission Directive 80/778/EC on water quality. Water for drinking and general domestic use, either hot or cold, should comply with this standard; generally such water is described as potable or wholesome.

2.11   It is exceptional for a water supply, either public or private, to be entirely free from aquatic organisms and consequently it is important that appropriate measures be taken to guard against conditions that may encourage microbial multiplication. Legionellae, like other opportunist pathogens including *Aeromonas hydrophila* and *Pseudomonas aeruginosa,* are common in the environment and as such can seed treated water systems during construction.

2.12   Contamination of water systems by micro-organisms does not occur, only during construction, but can be introduced during refurbishment, repair, alteration or during routine inspection and sampling.

2.13   Hospital sites are generally large and often contain complex storage reservoirs and distribution systems similar to those operated by water companies. The water companies or other specialist consultant can assist with the design, specification, tendering and commissioning of such water systems.

Water supply hygiene

Northern Ireland: Health and Safety Agency for Northern Ireland Publication HSA 62

Scotland: Refer to SHTN No. 2 for detail

2.14   Disinfection in accordance with BS6700 should be carried out. Guidance on disinfection is also given in HS(G) 70. The disinfection of water has proved to be effective in protecting communities from the spread of water-borne diseases. Nevertheless, some outbreaks of disease related to treated water supplies still occur. To reduce the risk of such outbreaks, the design should minimise:

a. direct contact with the internal parts of water-pipes and structures by people, animals or birds;

b. backflow (back siphonage) of contaminated water into systems conveying potable water (mains and storage structures).

2.15   Measures to protect against back siphonage are set out in the Water Supply Byelaws Guide. The principle is that the design of piped water systems should be carried out in a manner which minimises the likelihood of contaminated material or water gaining access to those parts of any water service conveying potable water. All water from non-potable sources (rain, surface run-off water, private supplies, drainage of foul water) must be regarded as a potential source of pathogenic organisms.

Water treatment regimens

2.16   The regimen of water treatment chosen should be agreed by the infection control doctor (legionella) and the nominated person (legionella). The regimen should be of proven efficacy, and substances and products to be used in contact with potable water supplies must be listed in the current edition of the Water Byelaws Scheme's (WBS) Water Fittings and Materials Directory (WFMD).

2.17   Chemical conditioning systems which are used in conjunction with potable water systems should be selected very carefully. Addition of any substance must not cause a breach of any requirement in the Water Supply (Water Quality) Regulations 1989 (SI 1989 No 1147), and any system for introducing a substance must be listed in the current edition of the WFMD.

Northern Ireland: Equivalent provisions are proposed for Northern Ireland (Oct 93)

Scotland: The Water Supply (Water Quality) (Scotland) Regulations 1990 with amendments and SHTN2

2.18   Consideration should be given to whether or not the process kills only the organisms flowing through the equipment (leaving no residual disinfecting agent) or whether disinfecting agents are released into the water circuits.

2.19   To ensure that adequate filtration and/or reverse osmosis is used to provide a pure water supply free of contaminants for conventional treatment, chlorine may be used. Ultra-violet (UV), ozone or the release of metal ions are alternative methods of treatment, each with specific applications and effectiveness. Further care should be taken in water serving clinical processes, for example dialysis equipment.

2.20   Where process water is to be treated, including cooling towers or water circuits as part of a production process, it is advisable to ensure that the concentration of any chemical treatment is not harmful if the treated water comes into contact with operators or product, and that safe conditions are maintained.

2.21   Water treatment systems should be fail-safe and have sufficient instrumentation to monitor their operation. For example, UV systems should incorporate a UV detector so that any loss of transmission can be acted upon immediately.

2.22   Regular inspection and maintenance of water treatment regimens at intervals, including quarterly records of inspection and testing both of equipment and water quality, should be instituted.

2.23   Hot or cold water delivered to basins and baths should be considered potable and as such, monitored regularly for wholesomeness; the period will normally be quarterly. Where automatic equipment is used for disinfection it should indicate any change in the amount or concentration delivered into the water.

Water softening

2.24   Water softeners tend to trap microbes, organic matter and other debris. In a relatively short time a biological layer (biofilm) forms on the surface of the resin. Eventually, these bacteria and associated organic/particulate matter break through the resin bed and can be released into the softened water. Local conditions such as water flow and quality and temperature determine the rate and frequency of colonisation and breakthrough in any installation. Microbial colonisation of water softener resins cannot be prevented by continuous chlorination, as regular exposure to chlorine has a deleterious effect on the resin bed. Backwashing (regeneration) purges the resin by releasing biological material that passes into the waste water. Although not a biocide, sodium ions in the brine solution are toxic to most freshwater organisms including legionellae. However, backwashing is not 100% effective in killing bacteria and therefore there is a risk of contaminated water passing into the system. Water softeners subjected to daily or routine frequent backwashing will supply water of acceptable microbial quality if the construction materials are of a type listed in the WRc Directory and the brine tank is protected and cleaned in the same manner as cold water storage cisterns. Softened water cannot be considered to be wholesome and a separate tap must be installed for potable purposes upstream of the softener.

2.25 In certain circumstances reverse osmosis and filtration equipment may also release bacteria into the water system. They should be installed and operated in accordance with the manufacturer's instructions.

Quality assurance

2.26 The current issue of British Standards Institution (BSI) Quality Assessment Schedule QAS/25/253 should be used. It relates to the manufacture and/or supply of water treatment chemicals and plant and the design, specification, supply, monitoring and maintenance of water treatment programmes for building services. The water services within its scope are boiler feed, hot and cold water services, and water used for heating, cooling and air-conditioning.

Fittings and materials of construction

2.27 All materials, including pipe fittings, jointing materials and components associated with the installation of cold water services, must comply with water byelaws. To ensure that potability is maintained it is also recommended as good practice to apply the byelaws to hot water service systems. (The current WRc 'Water Fittings and Materials Directory' should be consulted for suitable materials.)

Scotland: Refer to SHTN 2

2.28 Any protective coating applied internally to cisterns should be listed in the WRc directory. It is essential that these coatings are applied in accordance with the manufacturer's instructions and that the required period for curing elapses before any cistern is filled with water.

Access

2.29 All designs should incorporate sufficient access to allow the procedures for the control of legionellae to be implemented.

3.0 High risk areas

3.1 In high risk areas such as specialty departments or individual room(s) in a general department area, it may be preferable to provide separate small-scale systems.

3.2 Additionally, local water treatment may be considered necessary. It is also vital that cold water should be maintained below 20°C.

3.3 Cold water services should be sized to provide sufficient flow, and should be insulated and kept away from areas where they are prone to thermal gains. Stagnation should be avoided. Special attention should be given to the maintenance and monitoring of these systems.

4.0 Cold water services

Storage

4.1   The quality of stored water needs to be preserved to avoid microbial contamination and other loss of quality. Special attention should be given to all cisterns, tanks or other devices used to store water. It is necessary to minimise stagnation and stratification of the stored water. Cold water storage capacity should be limited, and a reasonable rate of turnover must be achieved. Pipework connections to and from the storage systems should be arranged to encourage good circulation within the system. Storage of unnecessarily large quantities will result in a low rate of turnover and consequent deterioration in water quality.

4.2   Delayed action ball-valves may help in ensuring that stagnation is reduced.

4.3   Storage cisterns should be located to minimise heat gains. To restrict microbiological growth it is important that the temperature of stored water is kept as low as practicable, ideally not more than 20°C.

4.4   Wherever possible, multiple cisterns should be avoided as they are prone to stagnation. Where multiple cisterns, including multi-sectioned single tanks, are installed, the design should enable a balanced outflow to be achieved. There should be interconnecting pipework at suitable varying levels. The interconnecting pipes should be on the opposite side to the water inlet and outlet and preferably diagonally offset. The installation must permit the isolation (by valves) of individual cisterns or cistern sections for cleaning. It is also preferable to arrange pipework such that sections not required can be disconnected. Wherever possible there should only be one supply to multiple cisterns.

4.5   Every cistern must be provided with a properly-fitting cover and any pipe open to the atmosphere (for example the overflow) must be properly screened (see Water Supply Byelaws Guide). The material should comply with WRc recommendations. Cisterns should be sited so that they can be maintained. (See Figure 1, cold water distribution.)

Distribution pipework

4.6   The cold water systems when running should be designed to ensure that the temperature of all cold water outlets does not exceed 20°C. Pipework should be insulated and not run in hot ducts. The design should ensure that the heat gain from the point of supply (the water meter) to the outlets is less than 2°C.

4.7   The Water Supply Regulations permit cold water to be delivered at temperatures up to 25°C, although in normal circumstances it will be well below 18°C. Chilling of the cold water system is not considered necessary. All cold distribution pipework, mains and cistern downfeeds should be located to minimise heat gains from their environment. They should also be thermally insulated.

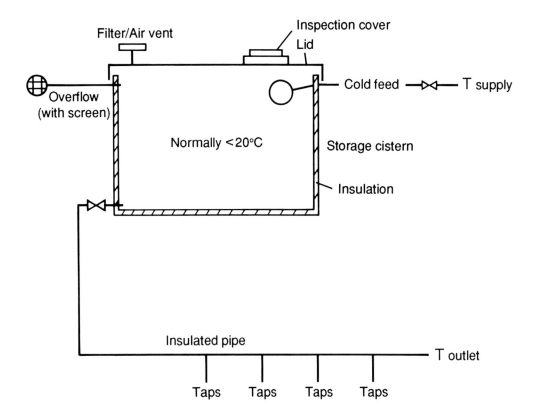

Figure 1: Cold water distribution – good

Cold water service pressurisation pumps

4.8   A pressurised cold water system will normally have two or more pump sets with a sequence control system. As the greatest risk is where water remains static, the control system should automatically sequence the pumps so that each operates at least once daily. The lead pump should be changed every week.

5.0 Hot water services

General

5.1   Generally this section applies to both vented and unvented systems and is independent of the method of heating the water. Similarly, the provisions apply to single-pipe or circulation systems.

5.2   The system should be designed to minimise the length of pipework that will contain water below 50°C. To prevent the colonisation of legionellae it is essential to follow the temperatures recommended. All the temperatures should be sustained under prolonged maximum continuous demand conditions (of at least 20 minutes) for which the system is designed. The installation of an orifice plate to measure system flows should be considered. Permanent continuous monitoring of temperatures via a building management system or data logger is recommended. An alarm system to indicate low temperature may be suitable on smaller installations. (See Figure 2, Hot and cold water services distribution.)

Cold feed cisterns and tanks

5.3   The requirements for the cold feed cisterns serving hot water service installations, when separate from cold water cisterns, are the same as for cold water cisterns given in paragraphs 4.1 to 4.5 above.

5.4   Some water authorities advise against the traditional practice of vent pipes discharging over cisterns. While it might be impracticable to re-arrange vents to discharge over a drain, any evidence of discharge should be investigated and corrected.

Calorifiers and water heaters

5.5   For the purposes of this guidance a calorifier is any device for heating domestic hot water. Therefore, these recommendations apply to all forms of hot water heating, including storage and semi-storage or high-efficiency minimum storage, vertical or horizontal calorifiers, or Angelery type heaters.

5.6   They may be heated by steam, or by high pressure hot water, or be direct-fired by gas, electricity, oil, coal or liquefied petroleum products. The application of the various systems is covered in HTM 27.

5.7   Vessels with dished ends should be specified. These should preferably be convex unless they are of the heated type with the heat source located beneath the concave base and designed to maintain temperatures in excess of 60°C. Unheated storage vessels with concave bases should be of a design which allows for the easy removal of any associated sludge.

5.8   Where storage calorifiers are used, the hot water storage capacity should be sufficient to meet the consumption for up to two hours; this must include the period of maximum draw-off. The installed hot water capacity should be sized for current needs and should not be designed with built-in capacity for future extensions.

Note: All pipes to be insulated

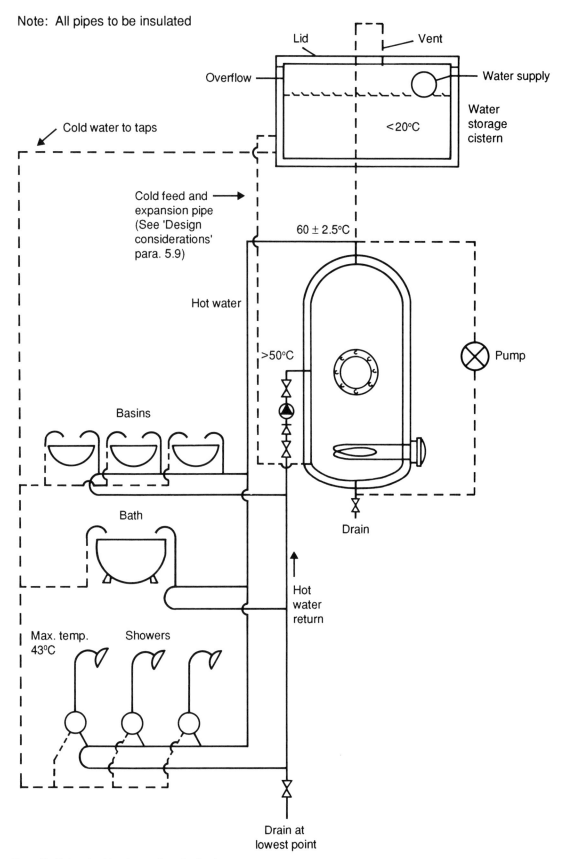

Figure 2: Hot and cold water services distribution

This will be achieved by setting the control at 60°C plus half the tolerance of the control device.

5.9 Traditional design practice has been to provide a non-check-valved cold-feed and expansion pipe to the storage cylinder and an open vent discharging over the cold-feed cistern. If a check valve is provided in the cold feed (to prevent warm water circulating in the pipe) it should be fitted within 300 mm of the calorifier. In such a case, the open vent should be arranged to discharge over a separate tun dish arrangement with visible Type A air gap sited at a level which takes account of the hydrostatic head of the system. This will prevent displaced water, on heat-up, discharging into the storage cistern. In addition the calorifier should be fitted with a safety valve of appropriate size.

5.10 The outflow temperature, under prolonged maximum continuous demand (at least 20 minutes) from calorifiers or other heaters, should not be less than 60°C. This applies to both circulation and single-pipe hot water systems. The positioning of the control and high limit thermostats, cold feed and return water connections must ensure that these temperatures are achieved.

5.11 Some devices are optimistically rated such that, at a continuous demand equal to their design rating, the flow temperature quickly falls below 60°C. Semi-storage or high-efficiency minimum storage calorifiers and instantaneous heaters are especially prone to this if under-sized. While it is acceptable that occasionally under peak instantaneous or prolonged demand the temperature will fall, it is not acceptable if this occurs frequently (more than twice in any 24-hour period) and/or for lengthy periods (exceeding 20 minutes). Under no circumstances should the flow temperature fall below 50°C. When the flow temperature does fall there will be a corresponding drop in temperature throughout the circulation system. It is recommended that disinfection is undertaken if the temperature of the calorifier falls below 45°C. The temperatures should be maintained 24 hours a day, seven days a week.

5.12 Where more than one calorifier or heating device is used, they should be connected in parallel, taking care to ensure that the flow can be balanced so that the water temperature from all the calorifiers exceeds 60°C at all times.

5.13 Calorifiers should be designed to minimise or eliminate stagnation and stratification. Legionellae multiply actively at temperatures from 20°C to 45°C. Stratification may occur in any calorifier or heater; the temperature gradient will depend on the rate of draw-off and heat input. In some calorifier designs it is significantly more pronounced and is a feature of their design. There will always be a layer of water in the temperature range that encourages maximum growth. It is not necessary to reduce the stratification in a calorifier during periods of demand.

5.14 Some semi-storage/high-efficiency calorifiers are supplied with an integral pump which circulates water in the calorifier. In other storage and semi-storage calorifiers, temperature stratification within hot water service heating vessels should be reduced by introducing independently pumped, time-clock-controlled circulation from the top to the bottom of the calorifier. It is important that this pump is only operated at times of low demand; this pump is often called the "shunt pump". The pumps should be run at least once per 24 hours for sufficient time to eliminate the temperature gradient within the storage vessel. To avoid the redistribution of "sludge", the direction and velocity of flow are important. The shunt pump may not be required if the return hot water circulation enters the calorifier at the same level as the cold feed and below the heating bundle.

5.15 There should be adequate access to calorifiers for inspection and cleaning.

Instantaneous water heaters for single or multi-point outlets

5.16 These devices usually serve one draw-off only and are either electrically or gas heated. The general principles and limitations of instantaneous water heaters are given in BS6700, Section 2. Basically:

a. the hot water flow rate is limited and is dependent upon the heater's power rating;

b. where restricted rates of delivery are acceptable, the heater can deliver continuous hot water without requiring time to reheat;

c. they are susceptible to scale formation in hard water areas, where they will require frequent maintenance;

d. this form of hot water heating should only be considered for smaller premises or where it is not economically viable to run a hot water circulation to a remote outlet.

Drains

5.17 All calorifiers and water heaters must be fitted with a drain valve located in an accessible position at the lowest point on the vessel so that accumulated sludge may be removed effectively from the lowest point. The drain should be of sufficient size to empty the vessel in a reasonable time (see Table 1).

Pre-heating cold feed

5.18 Pre-heating of the cold feed to calorifiers should not be used. The only time it is acceptable is when under all flow/demand conditions a temperature greater than 45°C can be guaranteed at the entry to the calorifier. Any pre-heater should have a low water capacity.

5.19 Where calorifiers are operated in series, the first is effectively a pre-heater. The design of the system should ensure that the flow from the first (that is, the feed to the second) is always above 45°C.

Distribution

5.20 Single-pipe and circulation systems should be designed to minimise the length of pipework that contains water in the 20 to 50°C range.

Circulation systems

5.21 The circulation pipework should be designed to facilitate balanced flows in the complete system. The minimum temperature anywhere in the circulation pipework should not be less than 50°C under prolonged maximum continuous flow conditions. While it is acceptable that occasionally under peak instantaneous or prolonged demand the temperature will fall, it is not acceptable if this occurs frequently and/or for lengthy periods. In a properly designed system it should not be necessary to use electrical trace heating to maintain the temperatures.

Table 1 Emptying times for calorifiers (approx)

Calorifier type	Diameter/length ratio	Capacity litres (galls)	Drain valve sizes mm (inch)		
			25 (1.0)	38 (1.5)	50 (2.0)
Horizontal	1:2.5	13,500 (3,000)	3hr 15min	1hr 30min	45min
		9,000 (2,000)	2hr 15min	1hr 00min	30min
		4,500 (1,000)	1hr 15min	30min	20min
		2,250 (500)	45min	20min	10min
		1,800 (400)	35min	15min	9min
		1,400 (300)	28min	12min	7min
Horizontal	1:1.5	13,500 (3,000)	3hr 00min	1hr 20min	45min
		9,000 (2,000)	2hr 10min	1hr 00min	30min
		4,500 (1,000)	1hr 10min	30min	20min
		2,250 (500)	39min	17min	10min
		1,800 (400)	32min	14min	8min
		1,400 (300)	25min	11min	6min
Vertical	1:1.5	13,500 (3,000)	2hr 45min	1hr 15min	40min
		9,000 (2,000)	2hr 00min	55min	30min
		4,500 (1,000)	1hr 10min	30min	20min
		2,250 (500)	38min	17min	9min
		1,800 (400)	31min	14min	8min
		1,400 (300)	25min	11min	6min

Times assume no hose and simple gate valve.

Notes: 1. Ball type valve(s) should be specified to avoid "clogging".
2. The drain from the gully should be of sufficient size to take the flow from the calorifier drain.

5.22   The design of the distribution system should be such as to minimise the length of any dead-leg. In particular, a hot water service return connection should be taken as close as is practicable to any draw-off (see BS6700). Spurs from circulation systems serving one or more outlets should not exceed 5 m. This length is measured from the centre of the circulation pipework to the point of discharge along the centre line of the pipe.

5.23   Any hot water service circulation pump should be installed with an appropriately sized and positioned non-return valve. In-line standby pumps should not be provided; this is to remove the risk of tepid water being maintained within a non-operational pump. A replacement pump, with any necessary jointing gaskets, should be supplied and stored adjacent to the operating pump so that in case of a failure, a quick replacement may be made. To simplify replacement, valves should be provided immediately upstream and downstream of the pump; any pump bypass should be removable. The standby pump and associated pipework should be disinfected before use.

5.24   Circulating pumps should be of adequate performance to ensure a minimum circulation temperature of 50°C. It is not permissible to shut down the pumped circulation system overnight. The position of the pump on circulation systems should be decided by the application.

Single-pipe systems

5.25 A single-pipe distribution system with electrical trace heating can avoid the problems of balancing the system and ensuring that the minimum temperature is maintained. Electrical trace heating of the self-limiting temperature type should achieve 55°C. Care should be taken to avoid cool spots within the system.

5.26 Where trace heating is used, dead-leg lengths, which should not exceed 5 m, are measured from where the trace heating ends. The trace heating should be connected to the emergency electrical supply. The continuity of the trace heat should be monitored to avoid localised failures.

5.27 Temperature alarms would also be advantageous (set to 50°C).

Blended water

5.28 The temperature at which water is generally used is much lower than the distribution temperature, and some form of blending is required. Water stored in the 25–45°C range encourages the growth of legionellae; therefore, particular attention should be given to ensuring that pipework containing blended water is kept to the minimum. Under no circumstances should it be longer than 2 m, provided that the complete length of the spur does not exceed 5 m. The same restriction applies to "communal" blending, that is, where more than one outlet is served by one device. For practical purposes, certain sanitary appliances with flexible shower hoses may exceed the 2 m overall length: 3 m would normally be adequate. This is acceptable provided the hose assembly can be detached for draining and if necessary cleaning. Again, the length is measured from the centre of the circulation pipework to the point of discharge along the centre line of the pipe.

Scotland: NHS EPM(93)3

Health Guidance Note — '"Safe" hot water and surface temperatures'

5.29 Central blending systems should not be used.

Space heating fed from domestic hot water systems

5.30 The domestic hot water system should not be used for space heating. This includes all radiators, towel rails, heated bedpan racks, etc, whatever the pipework configuration.

Unvented hot water systems

5.31 The possibility exists for stagnant water below optimal temperature to be held within the expansion vessel of this type of system, allowing legionellae to proliferate and contaminate the system. This risk can be minimised by incorporating the expansion vessel on the cold feed of the water heater/calorifier.

5.32 Designs of expansion vessels which ensure that there is a flow into and out from this vessel are not generally available, but such a design would further minimise risk.

5.33 Expansion vessels should be non-ferrous and compatible with the remainder of the system.

Strainers

5.34 Consideration should be given to the fitting of strainers and isolating valve(s) within the water pipework system to protect expansion vessels, thermostatic valves, etc against ingress of particulate matter.

6.0 Evaporative cooling towers

General description

6.1 The function of an evaporative cooling tower is to remove heat from a water circulation system. In process cooling, water is circulated direct from the cooling tower pond to the process equipment.

6.2 A more common application of a cooling tower is in association with an air-conditioning system where the cooling tower indirectly removes heat from a building, thereby preventing its occupants from becoming uncomfortably hot. Unlike process cooling cycles, water from the cooling tower is not used directly to cool the building's air-conditioning system. This is because, under normal summer design conditions, the cooling tower can only cool water to approximately 25°C minimum, and air-conditioning systems require cooling water as low as 5°C.

6.3 To provide the most appropriate temperatures for cooling requires a refrigeration process that absorbs low-grade heat from the air-conditioning system and transfers it as higher-grade heat to the cooling tower circuit at a temperature sufficient to enable evaporative cooling to take place within the cooling tower.

Water sprays and ponds

6.4 Heat rejection is achieved by circulating the water to be cooled through the tower. The warm water is discharged into the top of the tower through a set of open spray nozzles or a weir distributor. The nozzles are intended to spread the water over the full cross-sectional area of the tower and to cascade uniformly downwards. Immediately beneath the spray section is the "pack", sometimes called the "fill". The pack comprises a series of corrugated or latticed surfaces designed to provide a large wetted surface area. Water dripping from the bottom of the pack falls into the pond. The fan draws atmospheric air through the tower in the opposite direction to the flow of water. This contra-flow is the most efficient means of heat transfer but it also generates aerosols.

6.5 Materials used in the construction of these features should be WRc listed.

6.6 The distribution of water across the fill or pack is achieved by pressure jets as water sprays, or by trough and gutter distributors. The larger systems tend to have water sprays, since they more efficiently "wet" the surface of the pack. Spray nozzles are often mounted in grommets that should be of a type that does not support microbiological growth. (See Figure 3, Typical cooling tower installation.)

6.7 The pack provides a large wetted surface area which, in contact with the air flow, allows heat transfer by evaporation. It is essential that the materials used for the pack are non-absorbent. Particular care should be given to the design of the grid or pack support system to achieve free draining, so that pockets of stagnant water cannot remain after shutdown.

6.8 The pond collects and holds the water that circulates through the system and tower. The depth of the pond, the water level and the location of the

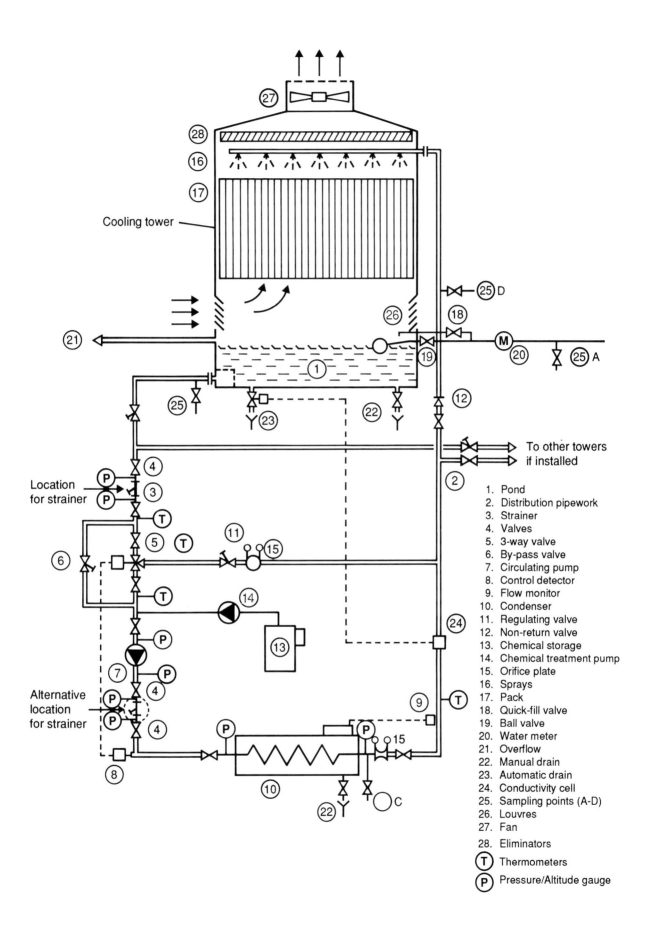

Cooling tower

Location for strainer

Alternative location for strainer

To other towers if installed

1. Pond
2. Distribution pipework
3. Strainer
4. Valves
5. 3-way valve
6. By-pass valve
7. Circulating pump
8. Control detector
9. Flow monitor
10. Condenser
11. Regulating valve
12. Non-return valve
13. Chemical storage
14. Chemical treatment pump
15. Orifice plate
16. Sprays
17. Pack
18. Quick-fill valve
19. Ball valve
20. Water meter
21. Overflow
22. Manual drain
23. Automatic drain
24. Conductivity cell
25. Sampling points (A-D)
26. Louvres
27. Fan
28. Eliminators

Ⓣ Thermometers

Ⓟ Pressure/Altitude gauge

Figure 3: Typical cooling tower installation

circulation water outlet should be arranged to ensure that air is not drawn into the circulation pipework either by vortexing or by any temporary drop in water level, for example when the spray or trough system above the level of the pond is filled on start-up. The water outflow pipe will usually contain a perforated cover plate to strain larger debris and help prevent the formation of a vortex above the outflow location.

Strainers

6.9   Since stagnant water can encourage microbiological growth, duplicate strainers are not recommended. Isolating valves should be installed each side of the strainer, and availability of spare strainer baskets will keep the plant shutdown times to a minimum. Where continuous operation is essential, and duplicate strainers cannot be avoided, each strainer should be capable of full system flow and the system should be operated with both strainers on-line. Temporary isolation of one strainer for cleaning will not significantly reduce the system flow. Manometer tappings should be installed across the strainer to allow operational checks for strainer blockage.

6.10   Sand filters should not be used.

Valves

6.11   Isolation valves are necessary throughout the pipework distribution system for the maintenance of three-way control valves, pumps and strainers, etc. The use of standard building services gate valves giving full bore when open and positive isolation when closed would be normal.

6.12   The bypass valve is provided for use in an emergency caused by failure of the automatic control valve. It is normally closed, and special care is needed to prevent water stagnation. It is preferable to have available either a spare control valve body or a T-section for the temporary operation of the system under manual control.

6.13   When a simple bypass arrangement is the only means of temporary manual control, use of a double regulating valve should be considered. This valve can be locked in the "cracked open" position, thereby providing a bleed through the branch that would otherwise be stagnant. Care should be taken at the design stage to ensure that overcooling of the water to the condenser does not occur.

6.14   Where three-way control valves are installed it is essential to have a regulating valve in the bypass circuit to allow flow balancing. Standard commissioning valves with locking devices should be installed so that the correct extent of opening, established at commissioning, can be reset.

6.15   The purpose of the non-return or check valve is to keep the pipework serving the sprays etc above pond level fully charged during control valve modulation and when the pumps are off. In practice, these non-return valves can tend to "let by" if not properly maintained and the cooling tower pond should therefore have sufficient free capacity to prevent overspill.

Pumps

6.16 To avoid stagnation duplicate pump sets are not recommended, therefore, replacement pumps/motors should be held as spares. The installation and pumps selected must facilitate rapid replacement to minimise plant downtime. Where continuous operation is essential, and duplicate pumps are necessary, the installation and controls should be arranged to automatically change over the duty pump twice weekly.

Water make-up, discharge and drainage systems

6.17 Evaporative cooling processes lead to an increase in the total dissolved solids (TDS) within the system water. The TDS concentration level is controlled by automatically discharging water from the system via an automatic dump valve to waste. Control is normally effected by means of a conductivity cell. When the conductivity level rises above a preset point the control system opens an automatic drain valve and allows water to discharge to waste. The drain should be located such that there is reasonable static pressure to establish flow, and the bleed line should be fitted with a regulating valve to allow precise control of flow.

6.18 This loss of water is then replenished with fresh water via the ball valve in the cooling tower pond. The ball valve should be set to maintain the cooling tower manufacturer's recommended water level. Incorrect setting of the ball valve can also allow escape of air and water droplets from the tower by unanticipated routes. The ball valve should always be at the opposite side of the pond to the water outlet to prevent air bubbles being drawn into the circulating water.

6.19 A conveniently located water meter should be installed in the pipeline feeding the ball valve to enable the maintenance staff properly to assess the system capacity and to monitor the quantity of "make-up" water. It is recommended that each pond should have a permanently fixed notice giving the volumetric capacity. This will allow the correct calculation of the necessary chemical dosage.

6.20 An adequately sized overflow should be situated a minimum 100 mm above the operating level of the pond.

6.21 On plant shutdown the relationship between the pond overflow and the pond water level should prevent any water draining back into the pond from the spray header distribution pipework.

6.22 The contents of the system must not be allowed to discharge into the surface water drainage, because chemicals used in the water treatment process may enter a watercourse and harm aquatic life or pollute the watercourse. Water from the cooling tower or circulation system must not be discharged into the surface water drainage system without the agreement of the local water sewage undertaking. Drains and overflows should be permanently piped to discharge above an open mesh trapped gully or a tundish with a clear air break to eliminate any possibility of back siphonage, and should be connected to the foul water drainage system.

6.23 A manual drain should be provided at the base of the pond. It should be of a size to enable the contents of the pond to be drained as quickly as possible, ideally within 30 minutes. Drains should be fitted to the low points of the distribution system to enable the entire distribution system to be drained within one hour. These drains should be a minimum of 25 mm diameter and of the full bore type such as a gate valve or plug cock.

6.24 Additionally, drains should be installed at equipment or localised low points to ensure that no pockets of stagnant water can be left within the system.

Air movement

6.25 Drift eliminators should be at the air discharge point to reduce the number of aerosols discharged by the cooling tower. It is essential that all drift eliminators are manufactured from non-absorbent materials. Drift eliminators should be of proven high efficiency and must be close fitting to prevent any air bypass of the discharge.

6.26 Louvres should be designed to permit free entry of air into the cooling tower and minimise loss of water by wind and splashing. The construction of the louvres must be such that pockets of stagnant water cannot collect on them.

Materials

6.27 Materials used in the construction of cooling towers should be non-corrosive, non-porous, resistant to chemicals and easy to clean. Certain synthetic materials, including some plastics and rubbers, are not considered suitable since they can promote the growth of bacteria. Natural materials, for example wood and cardboard, should not be used as these can be degraded by micro-organisms.

6.28 Suitable materials and fittings for use in the pipework distribution system which may also be applicable for the cooling tower are listed in the current edition of the Water Fittings and Materials Directory published by the Water Research Centre and will comply with the relevant British Standards. When fittings, materials and components become unserviceable or have to be refurbished, their replacements should be chosen from the relevant sections of the WRc Directory; BS6700 contains further advice. Where a material is not listed it must comply with the test methods specified in BS6920.

Other considerations

6.29 The pipework system should be installed according to good practice. It must include adequate draining and venting facilities and enough access points to simplify inspection and cleaning of the entire system. Sufficient disconnection points should be provided to allow dismantling for inspection and cleaning. Pipeline strainers should be installed to maintain "debris free" circulation water.

6.30 Altitude (pressure) gauges should be connected direct to the pipework, and not installed as remote reading gauges with lengthy runs of capillary tubes containing stagnant water.

6.31 Flow monitors are preferred to pressure differential monitoring devices because they eliminate the risk associated with pockets of stagnant water in the interconnecting capillary tubes.

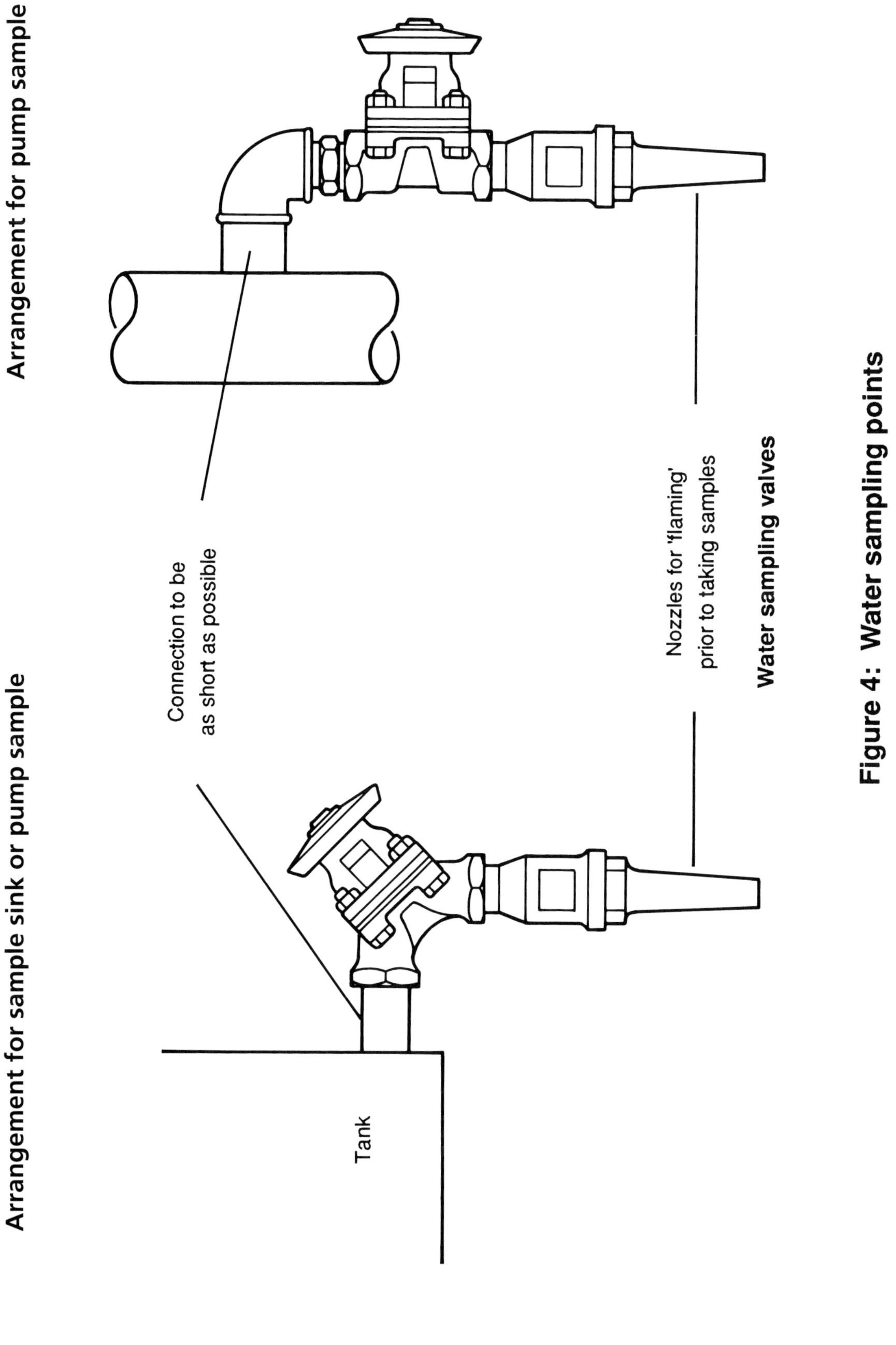

Arrangement for pump sample

Arrangement for sample sink or pump sample

Connection to be
as short as possible

Tank

Nozzles for 'flaming'
prior to taking samples

Water sampling valves

Figure 4: Water sampling points

Figure 4: Water sampling points

23

6.32   Sampling points should be provided to enable samples of water to be taken from the supply to the ball valve, the pond, the distribution circuit near the refrigeration machine and the point of entry of water returning to the top of the tower.

6.33   The sampling points should be located such that a 10-litre sample can be collected. The construction of the sampling point valve should be such that it can withstand the heat of a blowtorch that is applied to "flame" the nozzle before taking water samples. More recent improved analytical techniques are available which require smaller volumes. (See Figure 4, Water sampling points.)

6.34   Operational control of cooling tower immersion heaters should be introduced to avoid their continued function in mild weather and associated raised temperatures in ponds.

6.35   Where two or more towers are installed they should be connected in parallel and run hydraulically simultaneously to avoid stagnation. Stagnation in equalising pipelines between cooling tower ponds should be eliminated by the removal of the pipeline, ensuring no dead-legs remain. A common water level must be maintained to avoid problems associated with overflowing or air being drawn into the system. Consideration should be given to installing a larger section of pipeline between the two tower discharges to permit equalisation of water levels, and to modifying the ball valve so that one valve controls the levels in both ponds, nevertheless retaining the ability to operate towers separately, for example during cleaning.

7.0 Air-conditioning and mechanical ventilation

General

7.1   The design of the plant and selection of equipment within an air-conditioning or supply ventilation system should aim to minimise the distribution of excess moisture within the ductwork. The installation, and in particular the plantroom layout, should provide adequate access to items of plant for inspection and, when necessary, for affecting a cleansing regimen as part of the plant maintenance programme.

7.2   All materials used in the construction of cooling coils/chiller batteries and humidifiers should withstand bio-degradation; this applies in particular to surface finishes, mastics, gaskets, insulation, etc. Natural fibrous material should not be used.

Fresh air inlet

7.3   The fresh air supply inlet(s) must be located to avoid the possibility of air being carried over from evaporative cooling towers or being discharged from other extract systems and drawn into the system.

Cooling/chillers coils

7.4   The cooling coils/batteries and their components should be designed to allow regular cleaning.

Humidifiers

7.5   The cleanliness of the water supply is essential for the safe operation of humidifiers. Provision should be made for draining down supply pipework and break tanks for periodic disinfection and for periods when they are not required in service.

7.6   The addition of treatment chemicals for continuous control of water quality for humidifier/air handling units should be avoided. Consideration could be given to installing a UV system to control microbiological growth. Given the limitations of UV systems, however, this will require filtration to high quality to ensure the effectiveness of exposure of organisms to the UV irradiation. As with all water treatment systems the unit should be of proven efficacy and incorporate UV monitors so that any loss of transmission can be detected.

7.7   Overriding controls separate from the normal plant humidistat should be installed. Their purpose is to prevent excessive condensation when starting up. A time delay should be incorporated into the humidifier control system such that the humidifier does not start until 30 minutes after the ventilation/plant start-up. In addition, a high limit humidistat should be installed to switch off the humidifier when the saturation reaches 70%. This humidistat is to control added moisture; it is not necessary to install a de-humidifier to reduce the humidity of the incoming air if it already exceeds 70%. The normal humidifier control system should ensure that the humidifier is switched off when the fan is not running.

Spinning disk humidifiers

7.8   Providing the water supply is suitable, existing spinning disk humidifiers may be retained in service. When permitted by the local water authority, it is preferable that they be connected directly to a mains supply and not via storage.

Steam humidifiers

7.9   The humidifier lance design should prevent steam impinging onto the side(s) of the duct, condensing and generating excess moisture. Steam supply connections to humidifiers should be provided with a dirt pocket and trap set installed as close as practicable to the humidifier, so that the steam condition at entry to the humidifier is as dry as possible.

Ultrasonic humidifiers

7.10   The action of ultrasonic frequencies should not be considered an effective method for control of micro-organisms. The supply of water to the humidifier should be free from viable bacteria. The humidifier reservoir is accessible to micro-organisms, including legionellae, carried by the incoming air, and the water temperature in the humidifier during operation may be such as to encourage growth of these bacteria; biofilms may form. These units are capable of producing aerosols that may transmit legionellae.

System drainage

7.11   It is essential that cooling coils/humidifiers, fan scrolls (when necessary), eliminators and heat recovery systems are at a sufficient height from the floor to permit the installation of drainage pipework systems with access for maintenance.

7.12   Each device should have its own drainage trap.

7.13   A drainage/drip tray should be provided, to collect condensation on cooling coils (including the return bends and headers), and for humidifiers, eliminators and, if necessary, heat recovery devices. The drainage/drip tray should be constructed of a non-corrodible material and be so arranged that it will completely drain. To prevent "ponding" it is essential that the drain outlet should not have an upstand. The tray should be large enough to trap all the water produced by the device. Provision should be made for easy inspection of the tray. Any jointing material used to seal the tray to the duct must not be of a type that will support microbial growth. (The Water Fittings Directory lists suitable materials.) A slope of approximately 1 in 20 in all directions should be incorporated to the drain outlet position.

7.14   Drainage/drip trays should be connected to a drainage trap assembly that should discharge via a Type A air gap as laid down in BS6281:Part 1:1988. The depth of any trap should be at least twice the static pressure head generated by the fan so that the water seal is not "blown out" during plant start-up. (See Figure 5, Typical air-conditioning plant drain.)

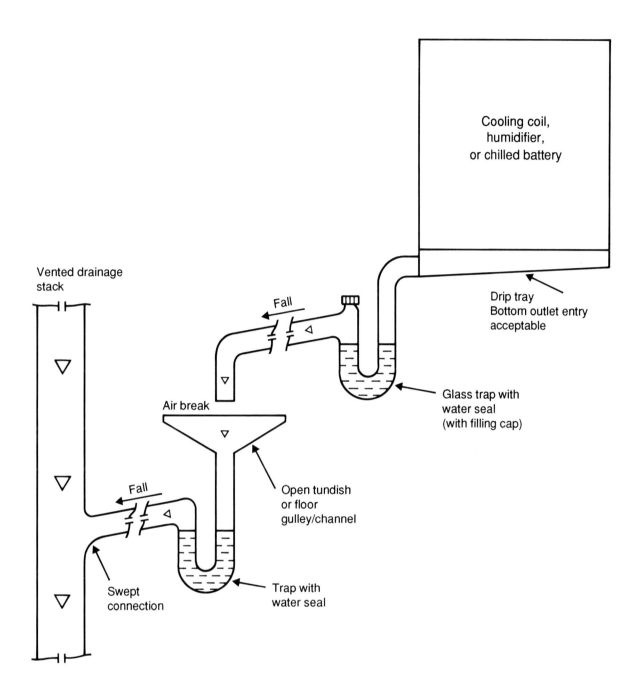

Figure 5 Typical air-conditioning plant drain

7.15 A trap need not be directly under the drainage tray if the pipework connecting the two has a continuous fall. Each trap must be of the transparent type to show (visibly) the integrity of the water seal, and should be provided with a means for filling. Permanent markers on each trap should be provided to show the water seal levels when the system fan is running at its design duty. Each installation should incorporate quick-release couplings to simplify removal of the traps.

7.16 If trace heating of drainage traps is necessary to provide frost protection, insulation should not be fitted, otherwise the trap will be obscured from view.

7.17   The pipework should have a minimum fall of 1 in 60 in the direction of flow. (Transparent pipework is not necessary.) Water from each trap should discharge over either an open tundish connected to a drainage stack via a second trap, or a floor gully (or channel). Where the drainage pipework from the tundish outlet, which should be ventilated, discharges into a surface water drainage stack or a dedicated plant drainage stack, the connection must be via an easy swept tee.

7.18   It will be necessary to disinfect humidifiers/cooling coils etc; thus it is preferable to discharge plant drains into the foul drainage system. The surface water drainage system may be used, for example when a plant is installed on the roof, but if chemicals are used during cleaning operations it will be necessary to discharge the effluent to the foul drainage system, for example by use of a hose.

7.19   The drainage system should be constructed of a corrosion-resistant material. It should be capable of removing all the moisture produced, for example during periods of maximum dehumidification load and in the event of full discharge from the humidifier during fan failure, and provide a means of safely disposing of the water via an independent drain. Drainage/drip trays for coils should be provided with a means to prevent air bypassing the coil (for example by the inclusion of suitable baffle arrangements).

8.0 Other design considerations

General

8.1   Legionellae may colonise other areas where droplets of contaminated water of a size suitable for deep inhalation are generated. Such aerosol-generating plant and equipment should not be installed next to patient accommodation. Some patients may be particularly susceptible to infection.

Hydrotherapy pools, whirlpool baths and whirlpool spas

PHLS WG Publication Hygiene for Hydrotherapy Pools (1990)

8.2   Hydrotherapy pools, whirlpool baths and whirlpool spas provide conditions that potentially favour the growth of micro-organisms including legionellae. Ease of maintenance should be borne in mind at the design stage and adequate water treatment included. Whirlpool baths which provide a single fill for each use do not present the same hazard as spas if the manufacturer's guidance for hot and cold water services is followed.

Portable/room humidifiers

8.3   Designs should not include the use of "portable" or "room" self-contained humidifiers (having a water supply that is sprayed/atomised into the room space). In clinical/patient areas the decision to use this type of humidifier must rest with the control of infection team.

Non-potable water storage

8.4   Non-potable water is sometimes stored for emergency use, for example, for fire-fighting purposes. These systems should be kept isolated from others by appropriate means that prevent back syphonage and microbial contamination.

Deluge showers

8.5   Deluge showers are intended for use in an emergency where a staff member or a patient has suffered external chemical contamination. Similarly there may be other special outlets used for personal emergencies, for example eye baths. These should not be installed on the end of lines and should be flushed regularly (weekly).

Trolley wash procedures

8.6   Trolley washing using high-pressure hoses is known to result in the generation of aerosols. The water supply should be taken from the potable system.

Lawn sprinklers and garden (or similar) hoses

8.7   In certain conditions, lawn sprinklers may retain stagnant water in the pipework/hose supplying the sprinkler head; they may also produce an aerosol spray. The pipework may be installed underground or via a flexible hose overground. In either case it is very unlikely that they can be completely drained down after use or when not required; at certain times in the year the retained water may be at temperatures suitable for the colonisation by, and multiplication of, legionellae. There is evidence linking cases of legionnaires' disease with permanently installed systems using underground supply plumbing.

Vehicle washing plant

8.8   Vehicle washing is carried out either using a hand-held pressure spray or by a "frame wash" which consists of a bay containing a rectangular pipework frame fitted with several high-pressure sprays. They should automatically drain down as far as possible after use.

8.9   Permanent hard standing for vehicle washing purposes should have an even surface to avoid ponding and have a slope or dish to a suitable drain.

Ornamental fountains

8.10   Ornamental fountains have been implicated in cases of legionellosis. They should not be situated under trees where fallen leaves or bird droppings may contaminate the water. Situations of exposure to high winds should be avoided as they can disperse spray beyond the immediate confines of the basin/pond. The apex of the water column/jet should not exceed the distance to the nearest edge of the basin/pond, for the same reason. An overflow/outlet to a suitable drain should be provided for easy emptying and cleaning. Where possible, a permanently installed freshwater supply pipe with topping-up device should be provided.

8.11   The installation of an ornamental fountain inside a healthcare building, for example a main entrance hall, is not recommended.

Ice-making machines and water coolers

8.12   Ice-making machines should be positioned so that their warm air exhaust does not impinge directly on taps or hoses supplying cold water. Legionellae can survive the ice-making process. These machines should not be located at the end of a branch.

Sanitary equipment

8.13   Hoses used with sanitary equipment such as "rise and fall" baths should be provided with quick-connector fittings to permit their removal for draining.

Automatic drain valves

8.14   Automatic drain valves for shower mixers and other mixers are not recommended. However, they are functionally desirable for bidets.

Cooling coils

8.15 Cooling coils for cold rooms and other refrigeration plant should have a tray to collect any water. The tray and its drain should be designed in a similar fashion to that for refrigeration plant.

Other publications in this series

(Given below are details of all Health Technical Memoranda available from HMSO. HTMs marked (*) are currently being revised, those marked (†) are out of print. Some HTMs in preparation at the time of publication of this HTM are also listed.)

   1   Anti-static precautions: rubber, plastics and fabrics*†
   2   Anti-static precautions: flooring in anaesthetising areas (and data processing rooms)*, 1977.
   3   –
   4   –
   5   Steam boiler plant instrumentation†
   6   Protection of condensate systems: filming amines†
2007   Electrical services: supply and distribution, 1993.
   8   –
   9   –
  10   Sterilizers*†
2011   Emergency electrical services, 1993.
  12   –
  13   –
2014   Abatement of electrical interference, 1993.
  15   Patient/nurse call systems†
  16   –
  17   Health building engineering installations: commissioning and associated activities, 1978.
  18   Facsimile telegraphy: possible applications in DGHs†
  19   Facsimile telegraphy: the transmission of pathology reports within a hospital – a case study†
2020   Electrical safety code for low voltage systems, 1993.
2021   Electrical safety code for high voltage systems, 1993.
  22   Piped medical gases, medical compressed air and medical vacuum installations*†
  22   Supp. Permit to work system: for piped medical gases etc†
  23   Access and accommodation for engineering services†
  24   –
  25   –
  26   Commissioning of oil, gas and dual fired boilers: with notes on design, operation and maintenance†
  27   Cold water supply storage and mains distribution* [Revised version will deal with water storage and distribution], 1978.
28 to 39 –
41 to 53 –

Component Data Base (HTMs 54 to 70)

54.1 User manual, 1993.
  55   Windows, 1989.
  56   Partitions, 1989.
  57   Internal glazing, 1989.
  58   Internal doorsets, 1989.
  59   Ironmongery, 1989.
  60   Ceilings, 1989.
  61   Flooring, 1989.
  62   Demountable storage systems, 1989.
  63   Fitted storage systems, 1989.
  64   Sanitary assemblies, 1989.
  65   Signs†
  66   Cubicle curtain track, 1989.
  67   Laboratory fitting-out system, 1993.
  68   Ducts and panel assemblies, 1993.
  69   Protection, 1993.
  70   Fixings, 1993.
71 to 80 –

Firecode

  81   Firecode: fire precautions in new hospitals, 1987.
  81   Supp 1 1993.
  82   Firecode: alarm and detection systems, 1989.
  83   Fire safety in health care premises: general fire precautions*†
  85   [Revision to Home Office draft guidance in preparation]
  86   Firecode: assessing fire risks in existing hospital wards,1987.
  87   Firecode: textiles and furniture, 1993.
  88   Fire safety in health care premises: guide to fire precautions in NHS housing in the community for mentally handicapped/ill people, 1986.

New HTMs in preparation

Lifts
Combined heat and power
Telecommunications (telephone exchanges)
Washers for sterile production
Ventilation in healthcare premises
Risk management and quality assurance

Health Technical Memoranda published by HMSO can be purchased from HMSO bookshops in London (post orders to PO Box 276, SW8 5DT), Edinburgh, Belfast, Manchester, Birmingham and Bristol, or through good booksellers. HMSO provide a copy service for publications which are out of print; and a standing order service.

Enquiries about Health Technical Memoranda (but not orders) should be addressed to: NHS Estates, Department of Health, Marketing and Publications Unit, 1 Trevelyan Square, Boar Lane, Leeds LS1 6AE.

About NHS Estates

NHS Estates is an Executive Agency of the Department of Health and is involved with all aspects of health estate management, development and maintenance. The Agency has a dynamic fund of knowledge which it has acquired during 30 years of working in the field. Using this knowledge NHS Estates has developed products which are unique in range and depth. These are described below.

NHS Estates also makes its experience available to the field through its consultancy services.

Enquiries should be addressed to: NHS Estates, Department of Health, 1 Trevelyan Square, Boar Lane, Leeds LS1 6AE. Tel: 0532 547000.

Some other NHS Estates products

Activity DataBase – a computerised system for defining the activities which have to be accommodated in spaces within health buildings. *NHS Estates*

Design Guides – complementary to Health Building Notes, Design Guides provide advice for planners and designers about subjects not appropriate to the Health Building Notes series. *HMSO*

Estatecode – user manual for managing a health estate. Includes a recommended methodology for property appraisal and provides a basis for integration of the estate into corporate business planning. *HMSO*

Capricode – a framework for the efficient management of capital projects from inception to completion. *HMSO*

Concode – outlines proven methods of selecting contracts and commissioning consultants. Both parts reflect official policy on contract procedures. *HMSO*

Works Information Management System – a computerised information system for estate management tasks, enabling tangible assets to be put into the context of servicing requirements. *NHS Estates*

Option Appraisal Guide – advice during the early stages of evaluating a proposed capital building scheme. Supplementary guidance to Capricode. *HMSO*

Health Building Notes – advice for project teams procuring new buildings and adapting or extending existing buildings. *HMSO*

Health Facilities Notes – debate current and topical issues of concern across all areas of healthcare provision. *HMSO.*

Health Guidance Notes – an occasional series of publications which respond to changes in Department of Health policy or reflect changing NHS operational management. Each deals with a specific topic and is complementary to a related Health Technical Memorandum. *HMSO*

Encode – shows how to plan and implement a policy of energy efficiency in a building. *HMSO*

Firecode – for policy, technical guidance and specialist aspects of fire precautions. *HMSO*

Nucleus – standardised briefing and planning system combining appropriate standards of clinical care and service with maximum economy in capital and running costs. *NHS Estates*

Concise – Software support for managing the capital programme. Compatible with Capricode. *NHS Estates*

Items noted "HMSO" can be purchased from HMSO Bookshops in London (post orders to PO Box 276, SW8 5DT), Edinburgh, Belfast, Manchester, Birmingham and Bristol or through good booksellers. Details of their standing order service are given at the front of this publication.

Enquiries about NHS Estates products should be addressed to: NHS Estates, Marketing and Publications Unit, Department of Health, 1 Trevelyan Square, Boar Lane, Leeds LS1 6AE.

NHS Estates consultancy service

Designed to meet a range of needs from advice on the oversight of estates management functions to a much fuller collaboration for particularly innovative or exemplary projects.

Enquiries should be addressed to: NHS Estates Consultancy Service (address as above).

Printed in the United Kingdom for HMSO.
Dd. 297562, C15, 12/93, 3396/4, 5673, 264319.